Antonio Garcia Dominguez
Kenia Milagro Piloto Tome
Mayelin Gonzalez Martines

Use of over-the-counter medications

Antonio Garcia Dominguez
Kenia Milagro Piloto Tome
Mayelin Gonzalez Martines

Use of over-the-counter medications

Risk of self-medication

ScienciaScripts

Imprint

Cover image: www.ingimage.com

This book is a translation from the original published under ISBN 978-3-659-65473-2.

Publisher:
Sciencia Scripts
is a trademark of
Dodo Books Indian Ocean Ltd. and OmniScriptum S.R.L publishing group

120 High Road, East Finchley, London, N2 9ED, United Kingdom
Str. Armeneasca 28/1, office 1, Chisinau MD-2012, Republic of Moldova, Europe
Printed at: see last page
ISBN: 978-620-8-27958-5

Authors: Dr. Antonio García Domínguez, M.D.

First Degree Specialist in M.G.I. and Gastroenterology

MSc. Integral Care for Women

Assistant Professor

Dr. Kenia Piloto Tomés

MsC. MedicalEmergency

Specialist I and II of Anesthesiology and Resuscitation

Assistant Professor

Mayelin Gonzalez Martines

Bachelor of Nursing

Assistant Professor

Introduction

Medicines are the most widely used health technology in the prevention and treatment of diseases at all levels of health care, and the ability of medicine today to interrupt or modify the natural course of diseases, to prevent them or, in any case, to make their burden lighter, depends to a large extent on them. The use of drugs is nowadays an everyday occurrence in the life of patients and the population in general, but their inappropriate use can become a real danger to people's health.

Self-medication can be defined generically as the self-administration, or administration on unqualified advice, of drugs to alleviate a symptom or cure a disease. [(1)]According to the World Health Organization, the term self-medication refers to the use of medicinal products by the patient to treat disorders or symptoms recognized by the patient or the intermittent or continued use of a medication prescribed by the physician, for recurrent or chronic diseases or symptoms.[(2)] This practice is a controversial issue, since there are those who reject it outright, arguing the damage that the indiscriminate use of medicines without medical guidance can cause to society; And those who defend it, arguing that it is the way to optimize and equalize health care for the entire population.

Historically, a medicinal substance, regardless of its origin or elaboration, has been understood as any consumable product to which beneficial effects on human beings are attributed. These medicinal substances, like today's medicines, were made up of one or more drugs, which are called the active ingredient or active substance [3] of these substances, to differentiate them from the non-medicinal elements of which they are composed.

In the Ebers papyrus, 1,500 B.C., we find a reference to the extensive use of substances for medicinal use in ancient Egypt.

In the first century AD, Dioscorides wrote De Materia Medica, a treatise with more than 700 substances used medicinally.

Since the most ancient civilizations, man has used products of vegetable, mineral, animal or, in recent times, synthetic origin as a way to achieve improvement in different diseases· [3] . Health care was in the hands of people who exercised the dual function of doctors and pharmacists. They were actually physicians who prepared their own curative remedies, some of them achieving great renown in their time, as in the case of the Greek Galen (130-200 AD). From him comes the name Galenic, as the proper way of preparing, dosing and administering drugs. In Roman culture, there were numerous ways of administering the substances used to cure diseases. Thus, electuaries were used as a mixture of various powders of herbs and medicinal roots to which a portion of fresh honey was added. The honey, besides being the substance that served as a vehicle for the active ingredients, gave the preparation a better taste. Sometimes sugar was used. A syrup was also used, which already contained dissolved sugar, instead of water and the whole was prepared forming a pasty mass. Galen made famous the great triaca to which he dedicated a complete work, and which consisted of an electuary containing more than 60 different active ingredients. Due to the importance of Galen in the Middle Ages, it became very popular during this period and was no longer authorized for use in Spain in the twentieth century. (4)

It is precisely in the Middle Ages that the pharmacist began his activity separate from the physician. In his apothecary's shop he made his magistral preparations, understood as the individualized preparation for each patient of the prescribed remedies, and they were grouped in guilds together with the doctors. During the Renaissance, a clearer separation of the pharmaceutical activity from physicians, surgeons and spice merchants began to take place, while a revolution in pharmaceutical knowledge was taking place, which was consolidated as a science in the modern age. The magistral formulation is the basis of pharmaceutical activity together with the officinal formulation, due to the birth and proliferation of pharmacopoeias and formularies, and this situation continues until the second half of the 19th century. (4)

From this moment on, specific drugs began to appear, which consisted of drugs prepared industrially by pharmaceutical laboratories. Thus, galenic forms did not acquire true prominence until around 1940, when the pharmaceutical industry developed and these began to be manufactured in large quantities. From then until today, the ways in which drugs are presented have evolved and the diversity that we find in the market is very wide. (5)

Polypharmacy, which according to the World Health Organization (WHO): is the simultaneous consumption of three or more drugs by the same patient, is in the senescent a daily occurrence as far as medical practice is concerned, being not only of scientific interest but also family and social; This is because with the growing number of geriatric patients, the horizons of diseases caused by drugs are widening worldwide, which today constitutes a problem whose magnitude is unknown in many countries[2] . This dangerous condition is already of concern to medical authorities at international level and is of interest not only at scientific level, but also at family and social level, since its collateral or adverse effects lead in many circumstances to an increase in hospitalizations, serious complications and sometimes, unfortunately, to death.

Drug utilization studies are an essential tool for the evaluation of the impact and the beneficial or harmful consequences of drug consumption by the community, which will enable health authorities to make correct decisions in the area of the management of available pharmacological therapeutic resources, as well as the analysis of the benefits, adverse effects and economic cost.[6]

Self-medication, both in industrialized and developing countries, is the most common reaction, and can be manifested by the use of natural medicine, stockpiling (saving leftover medicines), repeated use of prescription medicines, and direct purchase of medicines that should be dispensed by prescription.

It was not until after World War II that the value of drugs, considered as medicinal substances and their combinations or associations intended for animal or human use, acquired the importance it has today. The usefulness of some of them, such as antimicrobials in the treatment of certain diseases, contributed to the scientific community at that time turning its attention to the benefits they represented without taking into account the possible adverse effects they could cause. (7) Later, the scientific and technical development that has been achieved since then until today has allowed the number of drugs to increase from a few to more than 35,000 products. However, as the number of drugs on the market grew, two disturbing phenomena began to emerge, one biological and the other financial.

In the first case, the high number of adverse effects that began to be recorded, some of them serious, such as the case of thalidomide phocomelia, and in the second, the pharmaceutical industry began to mobilize large sums of money and became the second economic activity after the arms industry. In particular, prescribing errors and drug-related health problems are not a priority for medical students and general practitioners, despite the fact that this not only has a negative impact on the health of individuals, but also generates economic losses for patients and governments. (8-9) Drug-related problems account for 10-15% of the causes of hospital admissions. Studies have estimated the incidence of preventable adverse drug effects in the outpatient setting to be 5.6 per cent of all hospital admissions.

1 000 person-months· [10] The authors agree with Pérez Peña, [9] that drugs in contemporary society, and especially in health care systems, play four roles.

In the first place, they can be considered as tools, means used by health care providers to modify the natural course of a disease, prevent an illness or make a diagnosis.

They can also be considered as a way of measuring medical behavior; the use that prescribers make of this tool is evidence of their knowledge, skills, ethical and human values, and even their personality. On the other hand, drugs are also indicators for measuring the results of the impact that their use has on the community, as is the case with vaccines. Finally, it should be noted that drugs play a role in the doctor-patient relationship. This is the most frequent intervention used by the physician in his or her relationship with the patient.

In this line of thought, the World Health Organization (WHO) has recognized the need to establish a national drug policy and the importance of an associated research strategy that includes drug utilization studies.[2] These are promoted by this institution for the purpose of "describing the marketing, distribution, prescription and use of medicines by a society to determine the resulting medical, social and economic consequences".

However, for the physician, the focus of attention lies in the prescription and use of drugs by the population. Research on these topics produces new clinical therapeutic knowledge necessary to identify, according to the rules of the scientific method, the benefits of pharmacological therapeutics and also the health problems associated with the indiscriminate use of drugs, the occurrence of pharmacological pathology and to evaluate the potential effects of regulatory and educational interventions that originate from the research. They are of great importance in clinical research and of immediate transfer, or in the medium term, to the medical care· The therapeutic usefulness of a drug depends mainly on its ability to produce the desired effects with a minimum of undesirable effects tolerated by the patient.

Drug therapy should be based on the correlation of the actions and effects of drugs with the physiological, biochemical, microbiological, immunological and evolutive aspects of the disease. Underuse of the prescribed drug deprives the patient of the therapeutic benefits and overuse of the drug increases the risk of adverse reactions. It is therefore evident that drug utilization studies can contribute to the rational use of drugs. The rational use of drugs implies obtaining the best effect with the least possible number of drugs, for the shortest possible period of time and at a reasonable cost· Although it seems easy to achieve, practice has shown that drugs are rarely used rationally, one of the main reasons for this situation lies in the lack, in many countries, of reliable sources of information, based on the use of scientific research, on the use of drugs. The prescription of a drug is not an isolated act; it is part of a medical act and links the prescribing physician with other professionals, who are the ones who dispense and administer the drug, and again with the patient himself, who is the one who receives it. The errors that occur in this chain are potentially harmful to the patient and should therefore be prevented, avoided and corrected. The harm caused by these errors is caused by the administration or non-administration of the right drug, by the toxic effects generated by the drugs or by the absence of the expected benefit, and is linked to the wrong dosage or route of administration. To all this must be added the economic cost of the drug and everything necessary to correct the harm it causes.

Preventing and avoiding errors in the prescription and use of drugs is the obligation of all professionals involved in patient care and also of the healthcare institutions that must provide the means to prevent them, but it is a requirement, above all, of the prescribing physician.

The chairman of the editorial board of the British Journal of Clinical Pharmacology, Aronson JK, has defined a prescription as "a written order that includes detailed instructions as to what drug should be given, to whom, in what formulation and dose, by what route, when, how often and for how long.[(11)] This definition is considered to be very apt; prescription is not the end, but the

beginning of a process, as well as pointing out the uncertainty that accompanies the act of instituting a treatment.
This type of study will undoubtedly lead to new knowledge about drug-related problems.

Figueroa and his research team[9] identified that self-medication is mainly indicated in pharmacies.

Nowadays, it is demanded that physicians and other professionals in the medical field comply with their obligation to inform users about health services, and that the subject of the use of drugs be included in health education programs, an action that is not frequent in this environment. As stated,[2] the World Health Organization (WHO) has defined an adverse drug reaction (ADR) as any unintended or undesired effect resulting from the administration of a drug or medicine for diagnostic, prophylactic or treatment purposes, at doses normally used in humans.

It has now been found that the consumption of antibiotics throughout practically the entire world is very high, far beyond what is dictated by the norms of rational treatment of infectious diseases in humans.

This high consumption has important consequences on human health. It is also a global problem, a real threat to public health throughout the world. One of the most relevant consequences is the increase in the resistance of microorganisms (particularly bacteria) to antibiotics, i.e. the loss of their effectiveness in treating infections.

Every year on November 18, the European Centre for Disease Prevention and Control (ECDC) carries out an awareness campaign aimed at professionals, institutions, authorities and the general public in all European Union countries with the objective of achieving a more prudent use of these drugs and reducing their unnecessary consumption.·[12]

In Spain, the Ministry of Health, Social Services and Equality, along with other European countries, is developing activities for the rational and prudent use of antibiotics. [12]

Scientific entities have promoted numerous studies and publications with the same objective.

Other countries such as the United States, Canada and Australia support the objective and celebration of the *European Day for the Prudent Use of Antibiotics*. [12]

It was after the thalidomide disaster that the world became aware of the danger of using drugs without a surveillance system. In 1970, the WHO established as part of its programs and objectives to ensure the safety of medicines [2] , thus giving rise to pharmacovigilance, which is responsible for the study and post-marketing evaluation of the acute and chronic effects of pharmacological treatments on the population.

The information obtained from various studies shows that

suspected adverse drug reactions are currently an emerging pathology, with a high healthcare and economic impact. Results published by the journal JAMA on a compilation of 39 prospective studies, carried out in the USA over a period of 32 years in hospitals, show that ADRs account for 15% of hospital admissions, 6.7% of which are serious and 0.32% fatal. Recent data indicate that 100,000 Americans die each year from AMR, one of the six leading causes of death in the USA, and 1.5 million are hospitalized. (13)Other studies estimate that ADRs cause between 0.86 and 3.9% of emergency department visits and are responsible for 0.5 to 0.9% of mortality in hospitalized patients. (13)

Cuba has an age profile very similar to that of the developed countries of the world; at the present time it is among the oldest countries in Latin America and the Caribbean, but in two or three decades it will be the oldest. Currently, life expectancy at birth is 77.97 years and geriatric life expectancy is 22.09 years. (14)

The state of health of the adult is influenced by the natural and family environment, the degree of social life and daily activity, but illness and above all pharmacological therapy are aspects to which we must pay special attention for a better aging, with a good state of physical and mental well-being.

The aging process of the population has led to an increase in chronic and disabling diseases, which limit the activities of daily living, not only because of the consequences derived from the increase in their number, but also because of the high consumption of medications involved, which increases the risk of hospital admissions and the development of dependence.

Multiple studies have shown that comorbidity (concurrent presence of two or more medically diagnosed diseases in the same individual), daily consumption of four or more drugs, called polypharmacy, and disability independently increase health care needs, service utilization, increase costs, and have serious prognostic consequences for the elderly.· [15]

Primary health care is the first and fundamental link to guarantee a satisfactory aging process, to ensure a rational use of medications, to prolong life and to give life to the years with mental and physical independence.

In spite of the fact that numerous studies have demonstrated the high complexity of the inadequate consumption of medicines, as well as the consequences that this entails, there is no evidence of statistical data on the behavior of self-medication in middle-aged adults in our municipality, although it can be affirmed that consumption is high according to the data collected in our survey.

In view of the above, it suggests the following **research problem:** What are the results of the application of an educational intervention strategy for the control of self-medication in middle-aged adults?

Theoretical foundation or conceptual framework

A drug is a bioactive molecule that, by virtue of its structure and chemical configuration, can interact with protein macromolecules, generally called receptors, located in the membrane, cytoplasm or nucleus of a cell, giving rise to an action and an evident effect. Enzymes are also considered catalytic receptors, since they are able to interact with ligands. In this case, the drugs (agonists), in this drug-receptor binding, almost always involve supramolecular bonds, i.e. not of a high-energy covalent nature (around 60 Kcal mol), but rather weaker and reversible bonds such as hydrophobic, Van der Walls or hydrogen bridges. In the design of new drugs, descriptors are currently used, which categorize a molecule by electronic, geometric, quantum, thermodynamic and connectivity aspects, which makes the use of computer tools in the design of reference structures or heads of series feasible.

The term drug should not be confused with the term drug, as this error comes from a misleading translation of -drug- from English, therefore -drug- is not necessarily a synonym of drug and this error is still observed in many pharmacology texts.

When the drug, which is the active ingredient, is presented in a specific pharmaceutical form, it is called a drug. This already includes technological manufacturing contingents, which will determine an adequate bioavailability and stability of that presentation. That is to say, good absorption in a period of time, and no chemical or physical-chemical degradation affecting its functioning in a living organism, that is to say, without impairing adequate absorption, to pass from the biopharmaceutical phase to the pharmacokinetic phase, which determines the successful arrival of a bioactive molecule to the biophase or site of action, at concentration levels that guarantee an effect. Today, the tremendous progress in proteomics and the consequent alterations that proteins can undergo in their tertiary structures mainly, open up new and suggestive avenues in the research of bioactive molecules to combat dangerous infectious agents such as viruses, bacteria and cancer.

This definition is limited to those substances of clinical interest, i.e. those used for the prevention, diagnosis, treatment, mitigation and cure of diseases[16] and the name toxic is preferred for those substances not intended for clinical use but that can be accidentally or intentionally absorbed; and drug for those substances of social use that are used to modify moods.

Drugs can be substances created by man or produced by other organisms and used by man. Thus, hormones, antibodies, interleukins and vaccines are considered drugs when administered in pharmaceutical form. In summary, for a biologically active substance to be classified as a drug, it must be administered to the body exogenously and for medical purposes.

Drugs are mainly sold and used in the form of medicines, which contain the drug(s) prescribed by a physician.

Medication is understood as the state under which a drug is presented for practical use for the consideration of the maximum therapeutic benefit for the individual and minimizing undesirable side effects.

A **drug** is the sum of a dosage form + packaging (packaging, labeling, cartoning, package insert).

The primary packaging is that packaging or any other form of packaging that is in direct contact with the drug or dosage form (blister, tube, bottle, etc.). Secondary packaging is the outer packaging in which the primary packaging is contained (case, box, package insert, etc.).

The pharmaceutical forms are the active ingredients plus the excipients. They are a semi-finished product in presentation:

- Liquids: solution, syrup, tincture, infusions, sprays, eye drops, injectable and parenteral infusion, extract, emulsion, enema, mouth wash and gargle.
- Solids: Powders, granulates, tablets, dragees, capsule, pills or homeopathic globule.
- Semisolid: Suspension, emulsion, paste, cream or ointment, ointment, gels, lotions, suppositories, ovules, contraceptive jellies and creams and liniments.

- Others: Nanosuspension, poultice, transdermal devices, sprays, inhalers and implants.

The trade names of drugs vary in many countries, even when they have the same drug, which is why the name of the drug is used together with the name of the drug. [(17)]

Drugs can be synthesized or extracted from a living organism, in the latter case, it must be purified and/or chemically modified, before being considered as such. The activity of a drug varies due to the nature of these, but is always related to the amount ingested or absorbed. For example, oncology drugs, which cure cancer, are known as *highpotent active ingredients* and are used in very small concentrations to cure a special type of cancer. Each of these cause many side effects and overdose can adversely affect healthy cells, such is the case with oxaliplatin, letrozole, cisplatin, anaztrazole, etc. [(16)]

Dispensing is the act in which the pharmacist delivers the medication prescribed by the physician to the patient, together with the necessary information for its rational use. It is an act of professional responsibility isolated in time, whose succession in each patient can generate a pharmacotherapeutic follow-up, described within the pharmaceutical care.

The pharmacist is in charge of providing the medication prescribed by the physician, when a prescription is required; or any other medication requested by the consumer or user, when a prescription is not required, and if he/she considers it appropriate and adequate for the patient.[18]

Any chemical substance of natural or synthetic origin that when introduced by any route (oral-nasal-intramuscular-intravenous) exerts a direct effect on the central nervous system (CNS), causing specific changes to its functions, which is composed of the brain and spinal cord of living organisms, is considered **psychoactive**. These substances are capable of inhibiting pain, modifying mood or altering perceptions. Some of the psychoactive drugs: cocaine, crack, methylphenidate (ritalin), ephedrine, MDMA (ecstasy), mescaline, LSD, psilocybin (psilocybecubensis or mushrooms), salvia divinorum, diphenhydramine (benadryl), amanita muscaria, paracetamol (tylenol), codeine, tobacco, bupropion, cannabis, hashish.

Addiction is characterized by dilated pupils produced by the consumption of a psychoactive drug. It is considered that a psychoactive substance generates addiction in its consumer when it generates abstinence syndrome when it stops being consumed. [19]

Dependence is when a psychoactive substance generates dependence in its user when it meets at least three of four requirements:

1. It generates withdrawal syndrome when it is discontinued.
2. They lead the consumer to relapse.
3. It is used for recreational purposes, not therapeutic.

4. It has the ability to influence changes in the normal functions of the consumer's mind.

Over-the-counter (OTC) or over-the-counter (OTC) medicines are medicines that do not require a prescription or medical prescription for their acquisition. [20]It is a category of medicines produced, distributed and sold to consumers/users for use on their own initiative. Over-the-counter medicines are a group of drugs intended for the relief, treatment or prevention of minor ailments with which there is extensive experience of use. They have been expressly authorized as such by the health authorities of each country.

In 1990, the World Health Organization adopted the following definition of OTC medicines: "... medicines whose delivery and administration do not require the authorization of a physician. There may be different categories for these medicines, according to the legislation of each country."[21]

Over-the-counter drugs generally meet the following characteristics:

- its benefits outweigh its potential risks;
- have low potential for misuse and abuse;
- consumers/users can use them for conditions they can recognize in themselves;
- can be properly labeled (have product information on their packaging or on the inside of the package insert);

- the intervention of health professionals is not necessary for its safe and effective use.

These products may be available only in pharmacies or in other commercial establishments, depending on the regulations in each country. Likewise, in Latin America, some countries (e.g. Colombia) [21] have campaigns to disseminate the difference between over-the-counter drugs and drugs that require a prescription or medical prescription for their purchase.

They are, as stated by the World Health Organization, one of the pillars of self-care: "what people do for themselves to maintain their health, prevent and treat disease";[22] within the framework of what is called responsible self-medication, in which the consumer/user treats his/her diseases or symptoms with drugs that have been approved, are available for sale without prescription or medical prescription, and are safe and effective when used under the established conditions. It is therefore a legal activity, but requires qualified and independent information in order to make good decisions.

This is different from self-medication, which consists of the acquisition of drugs that require a prescription or no prescription at all. Self-medication has both economic and health consequences. On the one hand, it can lead to higher costs due to intoxication. On the other hand, it could worsen an illness or generate a new one.

A **polymedicated** patient is a person with one or more chronic diseases who takes more than six drugs daily and continuously for a period of six months or more. This definition can change both in terms of the number of drugs and the time required for drug consumption, depending on the care program in each community. [23]

A **placebo** is a pharmacologically inert substance used as a control in a clinical trial. The placebo is capable of causing a positive effect on certain sick individuals, if they do not know that they are receiving an inert substance (e.g. water, sugar) and that they believe it to be a drug. This is called the placebo effect and is due to psychological causes.

It is clear that the placebo effect cannot cure any disease. Cancer, for example, is not treatable with placebos alone. The effects are only limited to alleviating relatively superficial symptoms and not to actually curing the underlying disease; unless the disease in question did not exist from the beginning and was only a psychological imbalance (later also psychologically compensated).

Hypothesis

Through the application of an educational and therapeutic program, we can reduce the habit of self-medication and increase the knowledge of adults between 40 and 60 years of age belonging to clinic number 16.

Scientific novelty

There are studies that have made it possible to identify the problems caused in adults with respect to the ingestion of drugs without prescription both in the world and in the country. It is a novelty in the area to be able to develop a research of this particularity when there is only evidence of general and descriptive observational studies.

This work is of vital importance to raise the health culture in the prevention of self-medication.

General Objective

To evaluate the results of an educational and therapeutic intervention on self-medication in adults between 40 and 60 years of age belonging to the family medical office number 16 of the San Cristóbal health area during the period 2015 - 2016.

Specific

1. Characterize the study group according to: age, sex, dispensary group and diseases they suffer from.
2. Describe self-medication in terms of: use of medications, type of medication, and time of consumption as well as the presence of polypharmacy before and after the intervention.
3. To assess pre- and post-intervention knowledge of self-medication in the study population.

4. Determine the degree of satisfaction with the treatment among the villagers after the intervention.

Methods

Research classification: Research Development X

Context of the research.

An applied research was carried out based on an educational and therapeutic intervention aimed at modifying self-medication in adults between 40 and 60 years of age belonging to the family doctor's office number 16 of the San Cristóbal Health Area.

Universe and sample.

Clinic 16 of the San Cristóbal health area has a total of 591 patients.

patients between 40 and 60 years of age constituted the study universe.

The sample of 103 patients was made up of those who met the inclusion requirements.

Inclusion criteria.

- Patients between 40 and 60 years of age dispensed at the medical office, permanent residents of the locality.
- Patients who agree to participate in the study with prior informed consent.

- With physical and mental capacities apt to answer the questionnaire and participate in the educational intervention.

Exclusion criteria:

Patients who are not between 40 and 60 years of age, who move residence, or who do not attend 70% of the planned activities will be considered for exclusion.

Operationalization of variables

The variables selected for the study were taken from the individual and family clinical history and from the interview directly with the patients, which are listed below, clarifying in each case the classification scale used.

Operationalization of the main variables used

Variable	Type of variable	Scale	Operational definition
Age	Continuous quantitative	40 - 50 years. 51 - 60 years.	Years Completed
Sex	Qualitative nominal dichotomous	According to biological sex - Male - Female	Biological sex taking into account sexual characteristic s
Dispensary Group	Qualitative Nominal Qualitative Polytomous	Group I Group II Group III Group IV	According to the data in Family Health histories and based on the classification established by the National Health System

			Group I (supposedly healthy) Group II(at risk) Group III(sick) Group IV(with sequelae)
Diseases	Qualitative Nominal Qualitative Polytomous	Arterial hypertension Diabetes Mellitus Bronchial Asthma Ischemic heart disease Hypocholesterolemia Others.	Taken from family and individual health records

Variables corresponding to drug consumption

Use of Medication	Qualitative Nominal	Does not consume medications (does not include vitamins or natural products). Use at least 3 on a regular basis. Use 3 to 6 for more than thirty days or as indicated by	Characteristics of medication use according to the indicators of the Geriatric Functional Assessment Scale.

		different physicians. Uses more than 6 medications. They self-medicate or do not keep track of the medications they take.	
Type of medication used	Qualitative Nominal Qualitative Polytomous	Analgesics Anti-inflammatory Antidepressants. Vitamin therapy Others	Specific treatment for your underlying disease or other medications (more than 2 times per week frequently).
Time of consumption of medications unrelated to the underlying disease.	Qualitative Nominal	Less than 1 month. From 1 month to 1 year More than 1 year	According to the applied survey and the time of consumption

Variables corresponding to the results of the intervention

Pre- and post-intervention knowledge about self-medication.	Qualitative nominal dichotomous	Sufficient and insufficient.	According to the results of the surveys applied before and after the intervention

			Sufficient (when answering at least 5 items) Insufficient (when 3 or less items are answered)
Degree of satisfaction after treatment modification	Qualitative Nominal	The changes are seen as positive and the company has been able to adapt to them. Considered positive but unable to adapt to the new treatment He considers that the changes have had a negative impact on his state of health.	The patient's opinion on the therapeutic policies implemented is taken into account.

Methodology of the work

First stage

In the first stage it was necessary to proceed to the explanation of the informed consent that was applied to each person surveyed, it was recorded in the individual clinical history following the original format (Annex 1). Once this was obtained, a general data collection form was filled out using the individual or family clinical history as well as in direct interviews with the patient (Annex 2) where the general data were recorded, in order to identify those patients who self-medicate, after which the sample was obtained to carry out the work with the self-medication forms.

The form related to self-medication (Annex 3) was filled out and applied to all the patients included in the research as part of the sample. An initial questionnaire on prior knowledge of the intervention was filled out (Annex 4). The knowledge questionnaires were carried out directly in the framework of the control and follow-up medical consultations or during home visits with the support of the nurse and directly with the project leader. The questionnaires were initially applied to a group of patients to assess their understanding and were subsequently analyzed.

Second stage

It began with the implementation of an educational and therapeutic intervention.

For the therapeutic intervention, the evaluation of all middle-aged adults (under the inclusion criteria) was programmed in consultation with specialists of the Basic Work Group and respecting their office attendance schedule, the nurse was in charge of the organization of the programmed consultation and guaranteed, together with the head of the research, that the patients would be summoned. During the consultation, the review of documents, evaluation and modification of the inappropriate use of medications that were not related to a basic disease, and the degree of satisfaction with the changes were carried out. The educational intervention was carried out in several 30-minute meetings (according to the program) using the office itself to carry out the activities, using afternoon hours due to the low number of patients and more feasible for working patients. It was organized by small groups belonging to the same CDR for better organization and to facilitate the work. We used teaching aids and graphic propaganda on the subject of self-medication in each of the meetings.

The intervention was evaluated by applying the final knowledge questionnaire (Annex 5). Those who answered 5 items correctly were evaluated as sufficient and those who answered 3 or less items as insufficient. A semi-structured interview was used to evaluate satisfaction and adaptation to the therapeutic changes implemented during the consultation (Annex 6).

Intervention design

Educational strategy: Consists of behavioral and communication procedures capable of modifying adult lifestyles.

The proposed educational strategy was developed with middle-aged adults during 4 weeks, divided by a weekly meeting carried out in the form of demonstrative classes and group dynamics, taking into account the need for at least 70% of their attendance. The methodology used in this strategy was based on its open and flexible, participatory, group, practical and experiential character; its objectives and foundations respond to the principles and values of popular education, democratic participation, organizational development, transformation and change of life.

The main objective of the process is linked to providing them with knowledge on the most relevant topics. During the intervention, the patients were able to analyze their experiences, critically recognize their actions, mistakes and obstacles in order to transform and improve their reality.

Intervention Objectives

1. To raise the level of knowledge of the risk of self-medication in adults between 40 and 60 years of age.

Work sessions.

First session.

Subject: Introduction.

Objectives:

1. Create an environment of trust.
2. Assess the expectations raised by the activity
3. Present the Program and Methodology to be followed.
4. To raise the current problem of self-medication in adults.

Second session. Training

Objectives: To deal with the most interesting topics related to self-medication in adults.

Topics to be taught

1. Self-medication and polypharmacy.
2. Main drug-drug interactions.
3. Lifestyle and exercise changes
4. Frequently used drugs and their interactions

5. Most common therapeutic policies

Third Session: Group Dynamics

Objectives: To demonstrate through assertive techniques the harmfulness of the ingestion of drugs.

The activity guide through examples or a real problem situation, simulated the undesirable effects of a therapeutic misused. Discusses the arguments that led to the adverse reactions.

Through brainstorming, have participants recall a similar situation they have experienced or known.

Finally, the activity was closed with a written letter renouncing self-medication and polypharmacy, which was written by a participant.

It was also proposed the elaboration of health messages elaborated by the patients themselves related to the topic on the basis of what was learned. Teaching aids and graphic advertisements were made to culminate the activity, which were placed in public places chosen by the patients themselves.

Statistical processing

All the data extracted were recorded in a sheet, tabulated and processed, using in most cases the distribution of absolute and relative frequencies. Contingency tables were prepared for the application of the chi-square statistical test, using the MICROSTAT automated system, to search for the dependence-independence relationship between the variables and McNemar to determine the results of the intervention, where 0.05 was taken as the significant level of significance.

The results were presented in tables and charts that allowed a better understanding and analysis of the results in order to compare them with the national and foreign literature consulted.

2. In addition to quantitative methods, other theoretical methods were considered for the study.

- Historical - logical: It allowed us to analyze the behavior of the problem from the international and national level to the municipal level.
- Analysis and synthesis: It made it possible to reach conclusions about the state of knowledge on the phenomenon related to self-medication.
- Induction and deduction: It allowed to logically obtain scientific knowledge and to establish the unity between the particular, the singular and the generated.
- Among the empirical methods, the questionnaire was used.

Ethical aspects

For the implementation of our work, all the available bibliography for this purpose was censused and the references for each topic were cited.

In the first part of the research, the family health histories on file in the family's medical office were searched in detail, without extracting them from the premises. The work was carried out solely by the research team mentioned above.

Patient names and addresses were not used in the available data, and the data obtained will not be used for purposes other than the study itself.

All patients and their families were asked to consent to participate in the research, guaranteeing the principles of autonomy and confidentiality.

Analysis and Discussion of the results

Age groups	Male		Female		Total	
	No	%	No	%	No	%
From 40 to 50 years old.	24	23,3	37	35,9	61	59,2
From 51 to 60 years old.	15	14,6	27	26,2	42	40,8
Total	39	37,9	64	62,1	103	100,0

Table 1. Distribution of adults in the mean age according to age and sex corresponding to CMF No. 16.

^{2} X= 0,0277 p = 0,8677

Table I shows the distribution of the study group, where there is a predominance of the female sex with (62.1%), over the male with (37.9%).The age group that predominates is the 40 to 50 years with (59.2%) for both sexes, followed by the group of 51 to 60 with (40.8%), for a total of 103 patients representing 100% of the sample. There is no association between age group and sex.

The International Research Center in the United States recently reported that the demographic behavior of the population in more than 30 countries was in favor of the female sex, predominating generically in relation to males, arguing these results in the general population due to the direct effect of the favorable living conditions and socioeconomic well-being in which women live, as well as the influence of risk factors such as smoking and alcohol, which have a higher incidence in men, and which have a proven negative effect on the health of the individual.[24]

Other scholars of the subject are based on the fact that the incidence of malignant diseases is higher in men than in women, which has justified the inversion of the population pyramid in terms of gender, with a predominance of the female sex. Women's greater concern for their health and estrogen protection has also been raised. [25]

Table 2. Distribution of middle-aged adults according to History of Illness that motivated consumption and sex. CMF No. 16.

History of Pathological Diseases.	Female		Male		Total	
	No.	% (N = 64)	No.	% (N = 39)	No.	% (N = 103)
Health history	4	6.2	2	5.1	6	5.8
Arterial Hypertension	59	92.1	26	66.7	85	82.5
Diabetes Mellitus	38	59.3	21	53.8	59	57.2
Ischemic heart disease	21	32.8	4	10.2	25	24.2
Osteoarthritis	12	18.7	3	7.7	15	14.6

Bronchial Asthma	15	23.4	9	23.0	24	23.3
Hypocholesterol emia	11	17.1	7	17.9	18	17.4

Note: A patient may be taking one or more medications for the same condition, or may have no disease or more than one disease at a time in this table was repeated as many times as the patient referred.

Table 2 shows the most frequent reasons for consumption, being arterial hypertension (AHT) the condition that caused the highest consumption, since we found patients who had one or more drugs indicated for blood pressure control, followed by diabetes mellitus, ischemic heart disease, followed by bronchial asthma, hypercholesterolemia is also one of the conditions shown in the table and affects the study population with a lower percentage. Joint pain is evidence of the presence of osteoarthritis and arthritis in these patients, although on a smaller scale as shown. We would like to point out that if we add to hypertension the cardiac conditions that were the cause of consumption, it is confirmed that cardiovascular morbidity has an important influence on the population, and in fact is the first cause of mortality.

In other studies related to personal pathological antecedents in patients between 40 and 60 years of age, results similar to those reported in my study have been reported, with non-communicable chronic diseases such as arterial hypertension, bronchial asthma, diabetes mellitus and ischemic heart disease having the highest percentage of incidence.(25)

Arterial hypertension is an important risk factor for the progression of chronic kidney disease and a predictor of the development of end-stage renal failure, so there is consensus on the importance of its adequate diagnosis and control in these patients. A very high number of patients are not diagnosed at the outpatient level, which implies a more rapid progression towards renal and cardiovascular complications. [(26)].

A study showed that only 11.2% of the cases studied were under control[(27)] , thus demonstrating that early detection and adequate management of this condition allows for better control of the disease. [(27)].

Diabetes mellitus (DM) is an important health problem in our society, representing a significant percentage of patients admitted to hospitals over 60 years of age. Moreover, DM is a disease that predisposes to cardiovascular, renal and infectious pathologies, pathologies that often require intensive care. Thus, diabetic patients admitted to hospital will present an increase in morbidity and mortality. [(28)].

In other studies it has been found that in the months of September to February there is a higher frequency of onset of diabetic disease than in the rest of the year, it is possible that this is due to an exogenous triggering factor or perhaps an infection of viral origin. Diabetics are twice more prone to coronary heart disease and stroke than non-diabetics, certain medications that lower blood glucose also raise cholesterol, which promotes the formation of atheromas. They represent 20% of patients with end-stage renal disease who are included in hemodialysis programs, and constitute one of the largest groups of blind people in the adult population. In addition, there is a close relationship between diabetic disease and arteriosclerosis, obesity and hyperlipoproteinemia, a timely diagnosis allows to attend and provide differentiated assistance to patients in an incipient stage of the disease, and thus prevent complications or malignant forms of presentation, since in the elderly the possibility of suffering from these chronic diseases is doubled.[29, 30] .

Table 3. Characteristics of drug consumption according to age and sex. CMF No. 16

Age group	**Consume daily**				**Eventual consumption**				**Total**	
	M	**F**	**No.**	**%**	**M**	**F**	**No.**	**%**	**No.**	**%**
40 a 50	16	31	47	77.0	8	6	14	22.9	61	59.2
51 a 60	13	22	35	83.3	2	5	7	16.7	42	40.8
TOTAL	29	53	82	79.6	10	11	21	20.4	103	100.0

^{2} X= 0,2799 p = 0,5967

Note: The category of "never consumes drugs" is not included because no cases have been reported.

The consumption of medications in any group depends on many factors, among which we can mention morbidity, drug availability and patient compliance with treatment, among other factors, which vary from one region or institution to another and according to the period in which the study is carried out. In our study, 79.6% of the adults consumed medicines daily, being the group from 40 to 50 years old the one that consumes most of them, with the female sex standing out with respect to the male sex, despite the fact that as age increases, deterioration increases, this fact may be related to the characteristics of our sample. Only 20.4% did it eventually. It can be said that there is no association between the age groups and the level of medication consumption. In some studies reviewed by us, we found that drug consumption is higher,[31] although in other cases it was similar to ours. [32]

The middle-aged adult community usually presents more than one medical problem for which they request therapeutic actions that promote their wellbeing, and in most cases this is intended to be found with the use of medication. This leads to a high consumption of drugs. High medication in adults has been demonstrated in several studies.

Table 4. Distribution of middle-aged adults according to sex and amount of medication consumed. CMF No. 16

Number of medications consumed on a regular basis	Female		Male		Total	
	No	%	No	%	No	%
Only one	7	10,9	5	12,8	12	11,7
2 a 3	33	51,6	22	56,4	55	53,4
4 a 5	21	32,8	9	23,1	30	29,1
More than 5	3	4,7	3	7,7	6	5,8
Total	64	100,0	39	100,0	103	100,0

Of the population studied, 53.4% used 2 to 3 drugs, with a higher number of women, a figure to be taken into account, since it corresponds to more than half of the total group surveyed (n=103), while only 5.8% reported taking more than 5 drugs. Of course, on specific occasions an individual may consume 4 or more drugs for irrefutable needs. We have previously mentioned the frequency of "multiple pathology" at these ages and many times this multiplicity concerns chronic non-communicable diseases that require perennial medication. Our position in this situation is not to include it within the concept of "polypharmacy". (33)

We all know the frequency and magnitude of adverse reactions that occur when drugs are mixed. Some of them lead to extremely important discomforts such as dizziness, gait instability, drowsiness and confusion that disrupt biological, psychological and social functionality, even up to gastrointestinal

disorders, as also pointed out by Gusney[(34)] and Pallow[(33)] in their respective case studies.
All of which leads us to think of an intervention strategy to reverse this problem.

Drug utilization studies are an essential tool for the evaluation of the impact and beneficial or harmful consequences of drug use by the community, which will enable the health authorities to make correct decisions in the area of the management of available pharmacological therapeutic resources, as well as the analysis of benefits, adverse effects and economic cost.

Table 5. Distribution of middle-aged adults according to sex and type of medication consumed. CMF No 16

Types of drugs	**Female n=64**		**Male n=39**		**Total n=103**	
	No	**%**	**No**	**%**	**No**	**%**
Hypotensives	48	75.0	21	53.8	69	66.9
Diuretics	26	40.6	7	17.9	33	32.0
Hypoglycemic agents	31	48.4	11	28.2	42	40.8
Bronchodilators	13	20.3	10	25.6	23	23.3

Antacids	5	7.8	6	15.3	11	10.7
Sedatives and Hypnotics	10	15.6	4	10.2	14	13.6
Analgesics	7	10.9	13	33.3	20	19.4
Antibiotics	12	18.7	8	20.5	20	19.4
Laxatives	2	3.1	1	2,6	3	2.9
Others	3	4.7	2	5.1	5	4.8

In the group of women studied, the most consumed drugs were: hypotensives for 75.0 % of the cases, hypoglycemic agents 48.4 %, diuretics 40.6 %, bronchodilators 20.3 %, antibiotics 18.7 %, sedatives 15.6 %, analgesics 10.9 % and laxatives with only 3.1 %.

There was coincidence when analyzing the results in men. In general, a significantly higher consumption of the following drugs was observed: hypotensives with 53.8 %, followed by analgesics with 33.3 %, hypoglycemic agents 28.2 %, bronchodilators 25.6 %, antibiotics 20.5 %, diuretics 17.9 %, antacids 15.3 %, and less frequently sedatives and laxatives with 10.2 % and 2.6 % respectively. Other studies differ in some aspects related to ours, showing that the most indicated groups of drugs were analgesics, followed by diuretics and psychopharmaceuticals, and that antidiabetics were also of great significance, a fact that differs from our casuistry. Aspirin and nifedipine were included in the medications reported by other authors. (31,32)

Table 6. Time of consumption of medications unrelated to the baseline disease according to age group. CMF No. 16.

Time of consumption	From 40 to 50 years old		From 51 to 60 years old	
	No.	%	No.	%
Less than one month	21	34.4	19	45.2
From one month to one year	33	54.1	21	50.0
More than one year	7	11.5	2	4.8
Total	61	100.0	42	100.0

According to the table that shows the time of consumption of medications not related to the underlying disease. It is evident that out of a total of 61 patients between 40 and 50 years of age, there are 33 patients who consume medications for a prolonged period of time from one month to one year. Similarly, with a total of 42 respondents, 21 patients between 51 and 60 years of age, consume medications, representing 50% of this total, it should be noted the importance attributed to it, since with fewer patients there is a high number of consumption. For other authors (35) 75% of the adult population receives more than one drug of any type, with the logical increase of adverse reactions, which can be attributed to incorrect medical advice, the lack of advice for prolonged treatments and the alteration in the proper administration of the drug by the patient, to which we can add that it is not only a doctor who prescribes on several occasions.

Patients' knowledge of self-medication before and after the intervention.CMF No. 16.

Level of knowledge about self-medication.	Prior to the intervention		After the intervention	
	No.	%	No.	%
Enough	95	92.2	103	100.0
insufficient	8	7.8	0	0.0
Total	103	100.0	103	100.0

$X^2_{McNemar} = 6.13$

The table shows the level of knowledge achieved by the patients in the study, showing that prior to the intervention 95 patients were able to respond sufficiently to the interview out of a total of 103, representing 92.2 %, this being a high rate, with a small group of 8 participants who did not respond correctly. After the educational intervention, a better result was obtained, with 100% of the total number of participants answering correctly. This result shows the fulfillment of the main objective of the process, which is linked to providing middle-aged adults with knowledge on the most important and relevant topics. Through the intervention, patients were able to analyze their experiences, recognize mistakes and obstacles in order to transform and improve their quality of life.

The present study made it possible to modify the knowledge of adults between 40 and 60 years of age, as well as to transform some of the risk factors that influence self-medication.

Table 8. Degree of satisfaction of adults according to sex after modifying treatment. CMF No. 16.

Level of satisfaction	Sex				Total	
	Female	%	Male	%	No.	%
Positive	53	51,5	27	26,2	80	77,7
Does not fit	7	6,8	10	9,7	17	16,5
Negative	4	3,9	2	1,9	6	5,8
Total	64	62,1	39	37,9	103	100,0

The table above shows the degree of satisfaction of the study population after applying the intervention and modifying the knowledge about self-medication that the adults in the middle age group between 40 and 60 years of age had. For this purpose, it was necessary to apply an educational strategy consisting of behavioral and communication procedures capable of modifying the lifestyle of the adults. It was carried out in the form of demonstrative classes and group dynamics with the objective of providing new knowledge on this subject. As a final result, 77.7% considered the changes proposed by the project leader to be positive and expressed that they were able to adapt to them, 51.5% were women and only 26.2% were men. On the other hand, 16.5 % agreed that the changes were positive but they were unable to adapt to the new treatment, 9.7 % were men and only 6.8 % were women. 5.8 % of the total under study considered that the changes had a negative influence on their state of health, 3.9 % were women and 1.9 % were men, for a total of 103 patients, of whom 64 were women and 39 were men.

Conclusions

When considering the relationship established between middle-aged adults and drug regimens, we should take into account the problems that may arise. The sample of this series was mostly represented by the female sex and the age group of 40 to 50 years, all belonging to CMF No. 16. We found that the most consumed groups of drugs were hypotensives, hypoglycemic agents, diuretics, sedatives, and analgesics, in the same order; it was evidenced that a large percentage of the cases consumed between 2 and 3 drugs, and in a lower percentage the group of more than 5 drugs. Among the personal pathological antecedents that motivated the consumption of medications, the most common were arterial hypertension, diabetes mellitus, ischemic heart disease and bronchial asthma, in order of frequency. The highest percentage of adults between 40 and 50 years of age consumed medications on a daily basis. Regarding the knowledge achieved, it was sufficient in 100% of the study population after the intervention was applied. The results were also satisfactory with the level of satisfaction of the patients and demonstrated in practice.

Recommendations

- ✓ Disseminate the results of the study among the members of the core working group.
- ✓ Maintain surveillance and control of the patients who participated in the study.
- ✓ Extend the educational program to patients who do not belong to CMF No. 16.

Bibliographic Review

García Milián AJ, Alonso Carbonell L, López Puig P, YeraAlós I, Ruiz Salvador AK, Blanco Hernández N. Consumption of medicines referred by the adult population of Cuba, year 2007. Rev Cubana Med Gen Integr [Internet]. 2009 [cited 02 Feb. 2014]; 25(4): 5-16. Available from:

http://scielo.sld.cu/scielo.php?script=sci_arttext&pid=S0864-2012

2. World Health Organization. AIDE MEMOIRE. Safety of medicines. Pharmacovigilance. First stage. Geneva: WHO; 2004 [cited 31 Jan 2015]. Available from: http://apps.who.int/medicinedocs/documents/s17808es/s17808es.pdf

3. Albarracín, A. et. al. 1984 *Historia del medicamento.* Vol. I. Ed. Doyma S.A. Barcelona. 99 pp.
4. Mª del Carmen Francés CausapéThe Medicine Collection.
5. Lastres, J.L. Director of the Department of Pharmacy and Pharmaceutical Technology. Facultad de Farmacia - Universidad Complutense de Madrid. on the web page of the Facultad de Farmacia y Bioquímica de laUniversidad de Buenos Aires.
6. Fernández Alonso María C. Abuse of the Elderly PAPPS Mental Health Group: 2010

7. (Downloaded on: 1-02-2016 ISSN 1727-897X Medisur 284 April 2014 | Volume 12 | Number 1)
8. Ministry of Higher Education. Resolution 132/04: Regulations for Postgraduate Education in the Republic of Cuba. Havana: MES; 2004.
9. Bernaza G. Theory, reflections and some proposals from the cultural historical approach for graduate education. Havana: MES; 2004.
10. Bernaza G, Lee F. Some reflections, questions and proposals for innovation from the pedagogical perspective of graduate education. Revista Iberoamericana de Educación [journal on the Internet]. 2004 [cited 3 Mar 2009] ; 34 (2): [approx. 6p]. Available from: http://www.rieoei.org/deloslectores/755bernaza.PDF.
11. Bernaza G, Lee F. Collaborative learning: an avenue for graduate education. Revista Iberoamericana de Educación [journal on the Internet]. 2005 [cited 3 Mar 2009]; 37 (3): [approx. 6p]. Available from: http://www.rieoei.org/deloslectores/1123Bernaza.pd f.
12. European Day for the Prudent Use of Antibiotics (accessed October 31, 2014).
13. De Frutos Hernansanz MJ, Lázaro Damas A, Llinares Gómez V, Azpiazu Garrido M, Serrano Vázquez A, López de Castro F. Adverse drug reactions in a health center. Aten Primaria 1994; 14: 783-6.
14. National Statistics Office Center for Population and Development Studies 2010. Aging, Public Policies and

Development in Latin America. Present Challenges, Future Needs. MINSAP: ONE; 2010.

15. Blasco Patiño F, Martínez López de Letona J, Villares P, Jiménez AI. The polymedicated elderly patient: effects on their health and on the health care system. Inf Ter SistNac Salud. 2005;29:152-62.

16. FDA U.S.food and drugadministration. "Definitions. *Federal Food, Drug, and Cosmetic Act (FD&C Act*). Accessed June 16, 2010.

NationalCancerInstitute. "Biologic drug." *Dictionary of Cancer*. Accessed March 1, 2008. "Substance produced from a living organism or its products; used to prevent, diagnose, or treat cancer and other diseases. Biological drugs include antibodies, interleukins, and vaccines. Also called a biological substance."
↑http://www.boe.es/boe/dias/2011/11/30/pdfs/BOE-A-2011-18788.pdf

17. Ministry of Public Health. Directorate of Medicines and Technologies. Cuadro básico de medicamentos y productos naturales. Havana: MINSAP; 2014. [cited 31 Jan 2015]. Available from: http://www.hospitalameijeiras.sld.cu/web_hha/sites/all/informacion/servicios/farmacia/Introducci%C3%B3n%20y%20anexos%20CBM%20Y%20PRODUCTOS%20NATURALES%20%202014.pdf

18. .Royal Decree 1718/2010, of December 17, 2010, on medical prescriptions and dispensing orders . BOE. 2011/01/20; (17):6306-29.

19. Díez Abad, Paloma. "Psicología Europa." Accessed June 24, 2015.

↑Vocci, F. J.; J. Acri; A. Elkashef (2005). "A drug development for addictive disorders: The state of the science". *American Journal of Psychiatry* (162): 1431-1440.

Barbero-González A, Pastor-Sánchez R, del Arco-Ortiz de Zárate J, Eyaralar-Riera T, Espejo-Guerrero J. Demand for prescription drugs without medical prescription. Aten Primaria. 2006; 37(2):78-90.

20. osep-Eladi Baños Díez, Baños, Josep-Eladi Baños Díez MagíFarréAlbaladejo, MagíFarréAlbaladejo, FarreMagíFarréAlbaladejoPrincipios de Farmacología Clínica: Basescientíficas de la utilización de medicamentosElsevier España, 2002 ISBN 84-458-1166-5

. About OTC drugs.

21. About OTCs. http://www.aqfu.org.uy/informacion/index.php?Id=88&Pdf=1&Lan=es

22. Villafaina A, Gavilán E. Polimedicación e inadecuación farmacológica.PharmCare Esp. 2011;13(1):23-9.

23. Walston J, Hadley EC, Ferrucci L, Guralnik JM, et al. Research agenda for frailty in older adults: towards a betterunderstanding of physiology and etiology: summary fromthe American Geriatric Society/National Institute of

Aging Research Conference on frailty in older adults. J Am GeriatrSoc 2006;54:991-1001.

24. Selva A, San José A, Solans A, Villardell M. Differential characteristics of disease in the elderly. Frailty. Medicine (Madrid) 1999.

25. Weiss CO. Frailty and chronic diseases in older adults. ClinGeriatr Med 2011;27:39-52.

26. Acelajado MC, Oparil S. Hypertension in the elderly. ClinGeriatrMed 2009;25:391-412.

27. ALAD guidelines for the diagnosis, control and treatment of type 2 Diabetes Mellitus. Latin American Journal of Diabetes 2013.

28. American Diabetes Association. Medical Management of Type 2 Diabetes. Alexandria, VA, American Diabetes Association, 2012.

29. 32- Ward WK, Beard JC, Halter JB, Pfeifer MA, Porte D Jr. Pathophysiology of insulinsecretion non-insulin dependent diabetes mellitus. Diabetes Care. 2012; 7:491-502.

30. Álvarez SR. Drugs in the elderly. T1. Havana. Editorial. Ciencias Médicas; 2001. 166-81.

31. Roca GR, Paz PE, Losada GJ, Serret RB, Llamos Sierra N, Toirac EL et al. Pharmacotherapy in the elderly. T1. 4th ed. Havana: Editorial Ciencias Médicas; 2002. 542-4.

32. Pallow RL. Drug combination and potential for risk of adverse drug reaction among community dwelling elderly. NURS Res 1994 Jan-Feb; 43(1):44-9.
33. Gusney M, Tallis R. Prescription of contraindicated and Interacting drugs in elderly patients admitted to Hospital. Lancet 1984;2:564-7.
34. Bliss, U.R: Prescribing for the elderly. BrMed J 283:203-6, 2003.

Annex 1.

Informed Consent.

Yo:(Pcte)
____
_autorizo

(Dr.)
____ to
use the

information received from me for research purposes and for the benefit of the adult population.

____________________ Patient Signature

Annex 2: General data collection

Name(s) and Surname(s):

____

1) Sex: Female. ____ Male. _____

2) Age.
40-49 years old.
50-59 years old. ___
60 years old. ___

3) Address: _______________________________________

Please answer the following questions

1) Do you suffer from any disease?

None______ More from two_____

A ________ Four or more ____

In case of affirmative answer:

Which one?

____

__

2. Do you take any medication? Yes ______ No ________

Mark with an X in which way: ____ Daily _______ Eventually

Annex 3. About self-medication

Name and surname ______________________________

Age _____ Sex __________

The following questionnaire is about the use of medications, please answer as you see fit.

1) What group of medication do you take as prescribed by your doctor?

a) ____ Medications to maintain blood pressure in adequate figures (antihypertensive).
b) ____ Medications for the symptomatic treatment of pain (analgesics)
c) ____ Medications for symptomatic treatment of various respiratory allergies (antiallergics)
d) ____ Medications to increase the frequency and amount of urine (diuretics)
e) ____ Medications for infections caused by a diverse and complex group of organisms (antibiotics).
f) ____ Medications to maintain adequate blood sugar levels (hypoglycemics).
g) ____ Medications to treat insomnia and depression (psychotropic drugs).
h) ____ Medications to treat constipation or to evacuate the bowel (laxatives).
i) ____ Medications used to reduce or neutralize gastric acid secretion (antacids).
j) ____ Medications that act on airway obstruction (bronchodilators).

2) Do you take any medications on your own?

Yes ____ No ____

a) According to the groups mentioned above, state which of them.

____

____

____

3). Please state approximately how long you have been taking these medications (unrelated to your underlying medical condition).

a) Less than one month. _____

b) From one month to one year. _____

c) More than one year. _____

Annex 4. Prior knowledge questionnaire Evaluation _____

From the following questions you should answer according to your knowledge of medication use.

1. Of the following alterations produced by medications, check those that you consider to be frequent.

_______Heart rhythm disturbances

______ Nausea and/or vomiting

______ Itching or itching

_____Disorders of vision, hearing, etc.

2. In case of any undesirable symptom after ingesting the drug you should:

_______ Use other medication

_______ Taking medications that eliminate symptoms

_______Send immediately to the attending physician.

Do you consider taking a lot of medications a problem for your health?
Yes----- No-----
Why?

For researcher use:

Sufficient (when they answer no less than 5 items)

Insufficient (when 3 or less items are answered)

Annex 5. Knowledge questionnaire after the educational intervention.

Answer true (v) or false (f) as appropriate.

1- ____ Self-medication can be defined as the self-administration, or administration on unqualified advice, of drugs to alleviate a symptom or cure a disease.

2- ____ When using long-term drugs, we should not be afraid of adverse reactions.

3- ____ Polypharmacy is the simultaneous consumption of three or more drugs by the same patient.

4- ____ In the event of an adverse reaction, the treatment should be changed to another pharmacological group without consulting the physician.

5- _____ The medical indication is the physician's order indicated for each disease with specific medications according to the condition.

For researcher use:

Sufficient (when 5 items are answered correctly)

Insufficient (when 3 or less items are answered)

Annex 6 Interview

Semi-structured interview on satisfaction with changes in the use of inappropriate medications applied to patients.

Name: (Pcte) ______________________________

Through the application of some questions we want to know how you feel about the therapeutic changes used. For this we ask you to be absolutely honest and to answer as you see fit:

a) Has your health improved?

____

b) Do you consider the changes in your treatment satisfactory?

Yes _______ No________

____

e) In what form?

____

Index

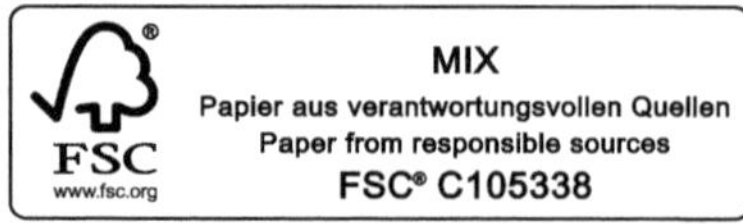

Printed by Books on Demand GmbH, Norderstedt / Germany